FOODS THAT

W9-APG-204

MAUREEN
KENNEDY
SALAMAN

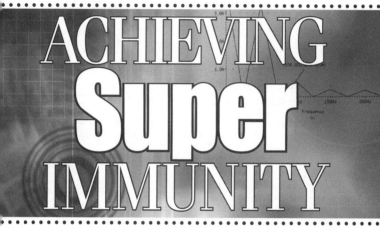

ACHIEVING
Super
IMMUNITY

Supercharge the Power Within to

Destroy Life-Threatening Diseases and

Today's Super Germs

STATFORD
PUBLISHING

IMPORTANT NOTICE

This book is neither a medical guide nor a manual for self-treatment. It is instead intended as a reference work only. The information in this book is meant to help you make informed choices about your health, but is not intended as a substitute for any treatment that may be prescribed or recommended by your doctor or health care practitioner. If you should suspect that you suffer from a medical condition or problem, you should seek competent medical care without delay

To Jorge Maumer—
As great a friend as any brother.

Achieving Super Immunity

Copyright © 2004
Maureen Kennedy Salaman
All rights reserved. No part of this book may be reproduced in any form or by any means without written consent of publisher/author.
ISBN 0-913087-25-4

Seventh Printing

MKS, Inc.
1259 El Camino Real, Suite 1500
Menlo Park, California 94025
www.mksalaman.com
(650) 854-3922 telephone
(650) 854-5779 facsimile

Distributed by:
Maximum Living, Inc.
20071 Soulsbyville Road
Soulsbyville, California 95372-9748
www.maximizeyourlife.com
(209) 536-9300 telephone
(800) 445-4325 toll-free
(209) 536-9375 facsimile

Scripture quotations are taken from the Holy Bible, New International Version®. NIV®. Copyright © 1973, 1978, 1984 by International Bible Society. Used by permission of Zondervan Publishing House. All rights reserved.

Literary development and interior and cover design by:
Koechel Peterson & Associates, Inc., Minneapolis, MN
Printed in the United States of America

CONTENTS

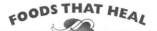
CHAPTER ONE

THE WONDER-WORKING POWER WITHIN

> *The rest of your life begins today—and what a great day it can be! The power you need to create anything you desire already lies within you.*
>
> —Stu Mittleman

DO YOU EVER WONDER how it is that some people sparkle with life and energy through the worst of the cold and flu season, and even the latest and the worst virus never seems to touch them? Have you known individuals who, no matter what their age, never get sick? What's their secret to not just keeping all kinds of diseases away, but for living in perpetual health? If you could find the answer to the fullness of health and wellness, even at the age of eighty, wouldn't you run after it?

The good news is that you need not run far,

for the secret lies within you. And there's even better news—the answers are not secrets at all. I'm here to tell you that there are basic principles that govern your body's immune system, and it's possible to strengthen and renew your internal defenses whether you're young or old. The secret is not in doing something to your body, but to help your body do what it was designed by God to do from the beginning. You can rekindle, replenish, and rejuvenate you today!

Perhaps you picked up this booklet because you've been frightened by the news of looming biological threats and reports of super germs, such as SARS (severe acute respiratory syndrome). Threats to your life and health exist at many levels, whether it is food poisoning, schoolyard epidemics of meningitis, the West Nile virus creeping across America, or biological terrorism in the form of anthrax or smallpox epidemics delivered through dirty bombs. You may have heard that something as ordinary as a sneeze in an elevator can transmit an incurable pathogen (disease-causing organism). It's scary, and it's true, and the media exploits it every day.

As we are faced with these serious health threats, conventional medicine continues to practice "crisis medicine"—waiting for symptoms to become life-threatening before making a diagnosis and attempting treatment. One gets the sense that they are forever chasing the latest problem, but never catching it in time and never getting ahead of the next crisis. Meanwhile, pharmaceutical companies are throwing up their hands in frustration because they can't develop new drugs fast enough to keep up with the chase. Ironically, they are partially responsible for the problem. The well-documented overuse and medical dependence on antibiotics, which actually educates stronger germs on how to defeat the immune system, lowers our defenses to a point where the plagues of old—chickenpox, mumps, measles, and whooping cough—are joining the new ones we hear about constantly.

What is the best way to protect yourself? By creating a super immunity within your own fortress, your body. Imagine having a police force inside your body that is always ready as a first line of defense to protect you from the many common and not so common bacteria and viruses you encounter every day. Imagine developing a super-charged immune system that has the strength to destroy the anthrax virus because your nerve system is functioning at 100 percent of its potential. It's possible!

God has made the natural provision within you to defend against these problems. All the antibiotics, vaccines, and medications in the world don't compare to the power He designed into your body through your immune system. He placed within you the thymus gland to be a powerful force for your body. Located high in the chest cavity behind the breastbone and extending into the lower neck below the thyroid gland, the thymus is equipping your body to battle against all invaders, repair damaged cells, and exterminate pathogens—twenty-four hours a day, seven days a week.

Here's how the thymus gland works. White blood cells called lymphocytes travel to the thymus and are changed into T cells by a substance produced by the thymus that is called thymosin. Those T cells, which are sometimes called "killer cells," exit the thymus and inhabit the blood, lymph nodes, and spleen, and from there they attack viruses, fungi, bacteria, cancer cells, parasites, and other harmful organisms. The lymph glands also aid in directing how many antibodies are needed and where they should go to destroy foreign cells. T cells are an extraordinarily versatile collection of specialized cells that make sure your B cells identify foreign invaders and enable the antibodies to mark them for destruction by macrophages that engulf and consume them. Antibodies remember invaders and quickly mount an attack when they encounter them again.

If your immune system is strong, your immune cells, organs, and fluids work together to recognize and stop the invaders from doing damage. This healing and germ fighting extend to the inside of every individual body cell, from the outer layers of your skin to the innermost stem cells in your bone marrow. We are truly "wonderfully and fearfully made."

But let me assure you that the wonder-working power created by a strong immune system won't come by way of eating fast food hamburgers, candy bars, and pop. Your immunity levels will never improve if your idea of physical exercise means not using the remote during evenings filled with television. So how do we supercharge our immune system?

This booklet will give you exactly what you need to champion your body's frontline of defense with strategies, herbal helpers, nutritional supplements, and fantastic foods. I will show you how to protect yourself against the extensive range of ever-threatening diseases through making your immune system become the strongest it can be. And I'll give you a clear understanding of what you need to protect yourself from, and how to accomplish it!

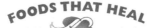
CHAPTER TWO

GIVE YOUR BODY A FIGHTING CHANCE

*Having good health
is very different
from only being not sick.*

—Seneca the Younger

IF SOMEONE WALKED UP TO YOU today and offered you 25 extra years of life . . . which they could prove would be delivered free of charge, how shocking would that be?

Well, that's basically what happened over the course of the Twentieth Century. An astounding 25 years of life was added to the average American lifespan through dramatic improvements in sanitation, and you and I are the fortunate benefactors. Most every home in America, rich or poor, has flushing toilets and running water. And whom should we thank for an extra quarter of a century of life? My answer may surprise you, but my thanks go to Henry Ford, and for good reason. Ford invented the assembly line and ushered in the mass production of cars, which led to the trucks that haul our garbage away. And nothing had a more profound impact on the quality of health in this land. So, every time you see a Ford on the road, think of the gift of 25 additional years and give thanks to Henry!

But while people are living longer, they are not necessarily living healthier. Instead of experiencing better health, the health of many people is deteriorating. While I cannot deal with the many factors that contribute to this general decline in health within the scope of this booklet, I want you to know that in your arsenal against disease, infections, and maladies, hygiene is the critical starting point in the battle. The word hygiene is derived from Hygeia, the ancient Greek goddess of health. It was the cornerstone of healing then, and it has not changed to this day.

When you faithfully do the basics of hygiene, such as washing your hands and keeping yourself clean, your immune system is free to concentrate its full powers against sickness. Not only is it important to practice regular hygiene, but you must watch for physical signs that your immune system is having trouble keeping up. The physical signs that we need to boost our defenses include thick cloudy mucus in the nose, weakness, fatigue, painful muscles, and fever. Fever is a classic sign that your immune system is being overwhelmed by the opposition, and it is a crucial time to intervene. I will show you how to battle these symptoms nutritionally in following chapters.

REDUCE BACTERIAL INFECTIONS
BY 90 PERCENT

The most common infections, including colds, are spread not through the air, but by the hands, specifically under the fingernails, to the nose, eyes, and mouth. A runny nose is your body's attempt to cleanse the waste. At the first sign of mucus going from clear to cloudy, it is time to act. Your body is being overwhelmed and is not able to cleanse waste anymore. Instead, it has become a storehouse for viruses and bacteria. Get rid of the mucus and you rid yourself of the bacteria, infection, and irritation that drain the strength of your immune system.

You can reduce your chances of getting bacterial infections by regularly following this procedure:

1. Keep your fingernails cut short and use a nailbrush. A recent University of Georgia study found that fingernails harbor 90 percent of the bacteria found on hands. The Centers for Disease Control and Prevention's hand hygiene guidelines recommend that natural nails only extend one-quarter inch past the fingertip. Using a nailbrush is effective in removing bacteria, but is largely ineffective with long nails.

2. Using liquid antibacterial soap to wash your hands, let the soap pour under your fingernails from the plunge spout. This way the liquid moves deep down under the nails where most of the germs are nesting.

3. Immerse your face in a basin of warm water

containing a small amount of the solution. Pretend you're an underwater swimmer and open your eyes in the water in order to flush the front of the nasal passageways and eyes.

4. Finally, blow your nose into a clean tissue, and repeat the procedure until there is no more mucus in your nasal passage. In this way, you slam the doors to germs.

HANDWASHING—A SOAPY SOLUTION

Less than 150 years ago, the unwashed hands of doctors were responsible for the deaths of one in four women in childbirth. Today, only one in 100,000 women die in childbirth, and surgery is infinitely safer primarily because of thorough hand-washing, which remains by far the most effective—and neglected—means of preventing the spread of infection. Admit it, your mother was right!

I know it's hard to remember to wash your hands. You're busy and don't have the time to stop at the sink and scrub those fingers. But I must tell you that if truly you want to be healthy, there is no substitute for anything less than squeaky clean hands!

Your choice of soap is far more important than you probably realize. What would you rather use, a scarred, pitted block of soap with dirt-filled cracks sitting in a pool of slime, or fresh soap out of a dispenser? Aesthetics aside, studies have found that liquid soap is more hygienic than bar soap. On a fresh bar, bacteria dies in 20 minutes.

But in the washroom, the bacteria stay alive for about 48 hours. And germs can be transferred from one person to another via a bar of soap.

Another important consideration is that most soaps contains propylene glycol, which is used in the antifreeze in your car and in professional garage floor cleaners. This cancer-causing ingredient is absorbed readily through your skin. I would never allow these cancer-causing agents in my body. Nor yours either. I prefer to use products that come from biblical sources, because I believe that God, through nature, knows best.

The soap you choose should kill germs and boost the skin's own defenses. Scientific studies have shown that the skin has its own defense system and is perfectly capable of keeping itself clean. That's why I developed the Eden Formulas liquid soap. It is a strong sanitizer with healthy nutrients and herbal scrubs, safe, natural ingredients, and preservatives. I formulated it with hawthorne extract, a bioflavonoid that has anti-cancer properties, increases circulation, and is used in heart medicine. Another ingredient is comfrey, which contains the healing agent allantoin. Comfrey has wound-healing properties and is used to treat leg ulcers. No matter how often I use it, it never causes dryness and heals red scaled skin on my hands and body.

Keep an antibacterial cleanser and hand-wipes in your purse, wallet, car, and office, and use them throughout the day. For example, you can use them to wipe off door handles in public restrooms, ATM machines, and places where you are exposed to germs from other people. This is especially important when traveling. There is no need to become obsessive about hand-cleansing, but it is a very simple and effective way to protect your body against disease-causing particles.

SINUS FLUSH

Much like the recent SARS epidemic, Chicago's 1918 influenza epidemic killed 8,500 residents. There would have been more deaths had osteopathic doctors not used the sinus flush to treat patients. Infections from bronchitis to pneumonia start from the sinuses and drip down the back of the throat. As the viral and bacteria-laden mucus is trapped, it works its mischief on your bronchial tubes and lungs causing throat and lung infections. The sinus flush prevents this from occurring.

Here's what you do.

First, fill a hot water bottle with warm water. Add a teaspoon of salt and mix until the salt is dissolved. This turns the pH balance into a saline solution. Put the rubber tube in the water bottle and the water regulator, which is provided on the tube, and cut the exposed end of the tube at an angle. Lower your head parallel with the sink with your mouth open, breathing rapidly (this closes the glottis, preventing water from dripping down the throat). Take the angled cut end of the tube and gently insert it into your nostril, slowly letting the water go into the sinus cavity, flushing out all the filth from behind your nose and eyes.

Do this three times a day. You'll feel completely revitalized and refreshed. You'll notice the swelling around your eyes disappear as the air circulates through your newly cleaned, clear passages. You'll feel wonderful!

READ ON FOR THE WAY TO WELLNESS

The tools and means to be and stay healthy are available to you. In the following chapters you'll learn what you can do to not only minimize the chances of becoming sick, but be among those still standing and able to render assistance to the sick, when everyone else has succumbed to the latest bout of influenza or a bioterrorist attack. There is always a way to wellness by following simple, practical steps for boosting your immune team.

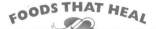
CHAPTER THREE

YOUR ANTIOXIDANT ARMOR

> *Nature is doing her best each moment to make us well. She exists for no other end. Do not resist. With the least inclination to be well, we should not be sick.*
>
> —Henry David Thoreau

IF I TOLD YOU that deep inside of you there was a barbecue pit shooting out sparks that burn everything they touch, you would think I was crazy. But there's a good deal of truth in it.

If you listen to the news, you've heard scientists refer to "free radicals" that, if not held in check, will decimate your immune system. Technically, free radicals are known as reactive oxygen species (ROS), in essence meaning excess toxic breakdown products of oxygen. Increasing evidence suggests their role in all disease processes. These molecular monsters use the very air you breathe, the ultraviolet in the sunlight on your face, illness, prolonged stress, and inflammation to ravage and destroy your skin, joints, tissues, organs, and bones.

They are what turns food brown, rusts metal, and ages your body, leaving their heavy footprints in the form of wrinkles, arthritis, heart disease, and other degenerative ailments. Essentially, free radicals are similar to sparks from a barbecue pit that puncture and damage cell membranes wherever they go.

Fortunately, in your foods and in supplements you have a suit of armor to protect you from their destructive effects: antioxidants. When your body is under attack by free radicals, during sickness, fatigue, or stress, you can fight back by eating foods high in antioxidants and supplementing with antioxidant vitamins and minerals.

The most effective antioxidant nutrients are vitamins A, C, and E (simply think ACE) and the mineral selenium.

VITAMIN A

There are many naturally occurring free radicals in your body and, due to today's proliferation of industrialized food processing and chemicals and poisons, an abundance of man-made free radicals that stress the immune system, especially the thymus gland. Vitamin A protects the thymus. Signs of a vitamin A deficiency include rough dry skin, poor wound healing, skin lesions, poor night vision, cuts that get infected, and ulcers.

When you are sick or injured and need additional support, take 20,000 Individual Units (IU) of vitamin A daily. Beta carotene, the nutrient that makes carrots orange, converts to vitamin A in the body. However, when you are sick, your body doesn't have the enzymes needed to convert beta carotene to vitamin A.

Vitamin A is so important to the immune system that virtually everyone with the HIV virus is deficient in it. Taking vitamin A while sick with the chicken pox can reduce the number of lesions. Vitamin A can also help the body recover from burns, strengthening the body's response to the injury.

Foods highest in vitamin A are orange-colored fruits and vegetables, such as carrots, yams, and pumpkin. One cup of carrot juice alone contains an incredible 24,750 IU.

Watch out for furtive pharmaceuticals interfering with your body's absorption of vitamin A. Strenuous physical activity within four hours of consumption, mineral oil, alcohol, iron supplements, and many drugs, such as cortisone, can block its absorption.

VITAMIN C

Vitamin C, or ascorbic acid, is the star player in your immune system. Smoothed on the skin, it acts as a sunscreen, blocking the free radical damage that contributes to skin cancer. When levels are low, the body suffers for it. Ascorbic acid deficiency has been associated with male infertility, duodenal ulcers, Crohn's Disease, and a decreased ability to fight off infection.

When you suffer a cold or flu infection, large amounts of vitamin C are used up. Because it isn't stored in or produced by the body, vitamin C must be supplemented continuously for therapeutic benefit. If you start supplementing during the early stages of an illness, you won't get as sick. As soon as you see thick, cloudy mucus, feel that sore throat, get the sniffles, or your muscles begin aching, begin your vitamin C protocol.

In order to achieve the therapeutic healing effect, vitamin C must be continually retained in the body. And since the body excretes what it does not immediately need, high doses must be taken at regular intervals throughout the day. Do this for one day only and establish how much you need. Begin with 5,000 milligrams. Two hours later take 1,000 milligrams. Continue taking 1,000 milligrams every hour—or 2,000 milligrams every two hours—and continue until you experience diarrhea or gas, then lower the amount to just below that. Your body will tell you how much it needs. This is the dose you need to make your body well. This is bowel tolerance, which for most healthy people means three to six grams (3,000-6,000 milligrams) a day. But when we are ill, our tolerance—and thus our body's need—may increase to 20 to 30 grams per day.

Always take vitamin C in a supplement formula that includes bioflavonoids, which will be described later in detail. In nature, vitamin C and bioflavonoids go together, forming the most potent form of defense against illness and inflammation.

Most people think oranges have the most vitamin C. Even orange juice doesn't have as much vitamin C as chili peppers, cherries, spinach, strawberries, broccoli, or cantaloupe. Even kale has more vitamin C than oranges. What food would you guess has the most vitamin C? It's papaya. One papaya has 187 milligrams of vitamin C. Compare this with an orange, which has a mere 80 milligrams. You can see from this, however, that if you need vitamin C for therapeutic value, you're better off sticking to the supplement form. Even if you like papaya, how many can you stand to eat in a day?

VITAMIN E

Supplementing with vitamin E is like having the Incredible Hulk as a personal bodyguard. Even conventional doctors (who long ignored vitamins) are taking notice. At a meeting of the American College of Cardiology, nearly two-thirds of the cardiologists in attendance revealed that they took supplements of vitamin E and/or other antioxidants.

Probably the most underestimated benefit of vitamin E is to the circulatory system. Since it acts as a blood thinner, it can help with cholesterol, heart disease, high blood pressure, and stroke. A deficiency of vitamin E can damage the red blood cells, nervous system, eyes, coordination, and heart arteries. Taking vitamin E can protect your

heart against the devastating effects of viruses and
protect your kidneys.

Foods high in vitamin E include wheat germ,
safflower seeds, sunflower seeds, sesame oil, walnuts, corn oil, hazelnuts, soybean oil, almonds,
olive oil, and cabbage.

SELENIUM

It is not enough to protect yourself from contagious illnesses, degenerative diseases, and free
radical damage. You need protection from injury
as well. The mineral selenium helps prevent the
inflammatory response that can cause so much
damage (and pain) to the body following injury or
illness. It is not usually the hit on the head that
kills, but the resultant swelling, pressure, and
bleeding of the brain that follows.

This is not the last time I'll discuss the dan-
gers of inflammation but, since it is the first time,
let me warn you that inflammation is now believed
to be the reason for chronic pain, heart disease,
Alzheimer's, strokes, and why normal cells become
cancerous. Many of the nutrients and formulas I
discuss in relation to immune-boosting: enteric-
coated enzymes, antioxidants and bioflavonoids,
are effective anti-inflammatories.

Selenium, a mineral and antioxidant, is particularly effective for rheumatoid arthritis as it increases
oxygenation in the synovial tissues in joint spaces,
where inflammation occurs. In one particular four-
month trial, selenium helped approximately 40

percent of a small group of rheumatoid arthritic patients.

A Chinese study showed that selenium at 15 parts per million added to table salt significantly reduced new cases of hepatitis B. And large doses of selenium markedly reduced the death rate from a viral hemorrhagic fever similar to Ebola virus. This study reported a reduction in the death rate from 100 to 30 percent. Ebola outbreaks in Africa have occurred in selenium-deficient areas. These facts are especially dramatic in light of the allegation that there is no cure for Ebola.

Selenium is high in seafood and foods grown in selenium-rich soil. But the amounts are so unpredictable that I recommend supplementation for optimum benefits. Make sure your supplemental formula contains at least 70 micrograms of selenium as L-selenomethione.

To protect myself against the effects of free radicals, I take and highly recommend Maximum Living's Antioxidant formula and Mineral Rich, which is their minerals in solution formula.

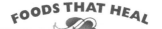

CHAPTER FOUR

BRAIN BOOSTING B VITAMINS

*Do not be anxious
about anything, but in everything,
by prayer and petition,
with thanksgiving, present
your requests to God.*

—*Philippians 4:6*

RECENTLY, a young working woman complained that she was anxious, depressed, irritable, and having trouble sleeping—the classic symptoms of stress. When I asked her what her daily diet consisted of, she told me she starts the day with coffee and a Danish, often skips lunch because she's "watching her weight," and then wolfs down a microwaved frozen meal for dinner. And she wonders why she experiences stress!

THE DAMAGING EFFECTS OF STRESS

Remember how, as a child, scary ghost stories made you feel ill? If you've ever felt the adrenaline rush of heat on your face, your heart thump in your chest, or the hair on the back of your neck rise, you've experienced the effect of stress on the body.

When you are frightened, nervous or anxious, your adrenal glands pump your body full of adrenaline (epinephrine) and noradrenalin (norepinephrine). These hormones are what make you dizzy, light-headed or suddenly forget that word you've been grasping for. It can be compared to revving up a car engine, then leaving it to idle at high speed. The most serious effect of elevated adrenaline, when persistent and unrelenting, is its damage to the heart and arteries. It beats down the immune system, leaving you less capable of protecting yourself against infection.

Chronic stress ever so subtly undermines both your nervous system and the serenity and healthful glow of your looks. When you are under stress your stomach as well as your other muscles tighten, preventing the villi from squeezing out stomach acid and impairing its absorption of nutrients, weakening your immune system, and flattening your color. As stress withdraws your body's stores of vitamins, minerals, enzymes, and essential fatty acids, it shows on your face, especially around the eyes. The plump collagen around your eyes thin, causing wrinkling and revealing dark blood vessels, which gives the hollowed-out look. Without adequate nutrients, your skin loses its luster and color, telling all who see you, including your image in the mirror, that you are losing the stress battle.

B VITAMINS BEAT BACK
THE EFFECTS OF STRESS

You can protect yourself against the nerve-jarring effects of stress and depression by taking a B-complex vitamin nutritional supplement and making sure you eat enough foods high in B vitamins, minerals, and essential fatty acids.

Due to their benefit to the nervous system, certain B vitamins are particularly valuable in protecting you against disease and infection. They are vitamins B12, B6, and especially B1 (thiamine). Although they must be taken with all the other B vitamins, they are worth noting here. Essential fatty acids, such as flaxseed oil and borage oil, will help protect and lubricate cell membranes lining the nerves so that you are better able to deal with stress. Flaxseed oil, in particular, is credited with reprogramming a faulty immune system, such as in autoimmune diseases and food allergies, when the body mistakenly identifies and attacks itself.

VITAMIN B12 AND A HAPPY HEAD

One of the ways that nature ages us is by reducing our ability to absorb nutrients. As you get older, you need to take B vitamins because your digestive system becomes less efficient. A lack of B vitamins can be caused by intestinal or stomach problems because chemicals needed for their absorption in the intestine are produced in the stomach. When you have trouble digesting food in the stomach or absorbing its nutrients in the intestine, the all-important minerals and B vitamins cannot be used by the body. This is so important that elderly people are often given shots of B12. Other symptoms that signal a need for B12 are a poor appetite, poor digestion, poor memory, poor coordination, depression, pale complexion, and intestinal disorders.

A lack of vitamin B12 (cobalamin) can produce psychosis, severe memory loss, impaired abstract thinking skills, mental confusion, delusions, hallucinations, and even brain and spinal cord degeneration (causing numbness). A Denmark study found low blood levels of the vitamin in one-third of hospitalized psychiatric patients suffering from depression and dementia.

One study showed how knowing a sovereign God made the difference between health, happiness, or taking the psycho-path through life. Dr. Lendon Smith showed a 70 percent rise in food absorption when people prayed before eating. This jumped to 80 percent when people held hands as they prayed. "Bless this food for our use." "Use" is the operative word here. Who would guess that our stress problem would be a lack of faith, resulting in a lack of vitamins? It puts saying grace for the food on our table in a whole new dimension.

B12 FOR YOUR IMMUNE SYSTEM TEAM

You need adequate amounts of B12 for your immune system team. In one study, after Japanese patients were given B12 for their pernicious anemia—a chronic B12 deficiency—they were found to have increased natural killer cell activity. B12 may help prevent cancer, evidenced by the fact that stomach cancer is high in those with pernicious anemia.

When elderly patients were given the pneumococcal vaccine, those with low B12 levels produced less antibodies. Their bodies were therefore less able to fend off the bacteria that causes pneumonia because they were deficient in vitamin B12. Studies have found that the AIDS virus progresses faster among patients with low B12 levels.

Foods high in B12 include liver, cold water fish, crab, Swiss cheese, eggs, and cottage cheese. Healthy food is essential to a healthy life, but in this day of imitation foods you have to be careful to avoid added chemicals and hormones. When eating seafood and meats, always buy organic so you know you're getting only nutrients. When buying fish, avoid those that have been raised in hatcheries or farms. Fish raised on processed food, usually corn, lack essential fatty acids, which are found in the wild. When you buy liver, always get liver from young animals, such as calves or baby chickens. Older animal livers are toxic with hormones and antiobiotics.

I am always conscious of getting the best possible value for every dollar spent on food. Confronting the burly butcher at a special chemical-free meat shop, I asked for a piece of beef with no fat and no bone. "Lady," came the gruff reply, "we've been trying to grow them like that for years, but they just fall over." What a comedian!

Here's a great recipe for liver (ugh!) from my book *Nutrition: The Cancer Answer II*. Even if I don't find liver palatable, with this recipe, you won't.

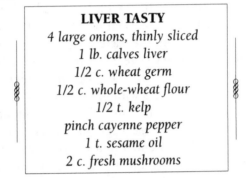

LIVER TASTY
4 large onions, thinly sliced
1 lb. calves liver
1/2 c. wheat germ
1/2 c. whole-wheat flour
1/2 t. kelp
pinch cayenne pepper
1 t. sesame oil
2 c. fresh mushrooms

Sauté onions until transparent. Slice liver into small strips 2" by 1/4" thick. In a dish or plastic bag, combine wheat germ, whole-wheat flour, kelp, and cayenne. Lightly heat extra virgin olive oil in a skillet. Coat strips of liver in the whole grain/wheat germ flour mixture and sauté lightly, rotating until all surfaces of liver are lightly browned. Do not overcook. After cooking liver, sauté mushrooms lightly in same pan. Combine mushrooms in pan with liver and sauté lightly. Serves six.

There are other B vitamins and nutrients important to your immune and mental health, and which should be included in any B-complex vitamin supplement.

VITAMIN B6

Vitamin B6 (pyridoxine) is remarkably similar to vitamin C in its ability to protect your skin from the ravaging effects of the sun. Combined with folic acid and zinc, it literally rebuilds DNA. One of the ways the B vitamins protect the nervous system is by making sure the cholesterol you need stays on the nerves and not on the arteries. Vitamin B6 and vitamin C work together to prevent allergic responses that causes the brain to swell. Vitamin B6 has helped with mood swings and the swelling associated with PMS and joint problems.

Vitamin B6 should not be taken alone as it can cause an imbalance or deficiency of other B vitamins. The more protein you eat, the more B6 you need, so if you are in the habit of eating meat at every meal, you should supplement with a B-complex formula. Foods high in B6 include brewer's yeast, brown rice, whole wheat and wheat germ, soybeans, rye, lentils, sunflower seeds, and walnuts. You needn't worry about creating an imbalance by eating these foods. God made our food perfect, with just the right combinations of nutrients.

THIAMINE

The next time you're out hiking in the woods, take along your thiamine, or B1. It may save your life. Lyme disease is spread by ticks, and West Nile Virus, a form of encephalitis, is associated with mosquito bites. If you're like me and prefer not to perfume yourself with bug spray, you need something that will keep you healthy but unattractive to blood-sucking insects. Thiamine may be the solution. It works for me, but it may not work for everyone. However, the anecdotal evidence is compelling enough to take a shot at it. Since thiamine is eliminated through the skin, it alters your scent, making you repulsive to mosquitoes and ticks.

Jonathan Yu, M.D., recommends 300 mg for adults, 150 mg for children, and 75 mg for babies. Bob, an Idaho fisherman, takes a B vitamin formula containing 30 mg of vitamin B1 every day, April through October. He finds it repels mosquitoes, black flies, noseeums, and gnats. He claims he hasn't had a mosquito bite in 33 years, but says it doesn't work on stinging insects.

Thiamine is found in brewer's yeast, wheat germ, bran, and blackstrap molasses.

SUPPLEMENTING FROM GOD'S GARDEN

If you could choose a food or supplement that would be the healthiest and most beneficial of all, what would you look for? First, it would be as close to the way God made it as possible. Every nutrient would be derived from natural sources, not synthesized. Next, it would include all the vitamins, minerals, and natural herbs that are needed for optimum health.

What else? What's missing? Food, of course! Food in a supplement? Yes, it's come to that. Do you eat fresh vegetables the day you buy them? Do you buy organic? If you don't, you're eating inferior produce. From the day they are picked from the ground or tree, fruits and vegetables lose nutrients. Who knows how much is left in that bag of carrots you bought a week ago?

The freshest, youngest food has the highest amount of nutrients. In plants, it is 1/4" seed sprouts. God made sprouts in their wholeness with the most potent forms of highly concentrated vitamins and minerals.

The most beneficial vitamin and mineral supplement on the market today is Maximum Living's Vita-Sprout. It has all the nutrients discovered to be beneficial today, including freeze-dried sprouts, vegetables, and herbals. And to make sure the entire complex of B vitamins are digested and assimilated properly, it includes friendly-body bacteria acidophilus, which I will describe in a later chapter. Nothing could be more complete for your immune system team than this power-packed, God-given formula.

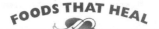
CHAPTER FIVE

THE SPARK
OF MINERALS

For six years sow your fields,
and for six years prune your
vineyards and gather their crops.
But in the seventh year the land
is to have a sabbath of rest,
a sabbath to the LORD.
Do not sow your fields
or prune your vineyards.

—*Leviticus 25:3-4*

WHY DO WE NEED MINERALS?

Let me illustrate why with a story. A friend of mine liked to bake cookies ahead of time for the holiday season and store them in the freezer. But her family always found them, and by Christmas not a crumb was left. One year she baked as usual and then put all the cookies in special containers before freezing them. This time not one cookie was touched. She had labeled all the containers "four cups sliced zucchini."

These days, with land at a premium and farm

equipment indebting the farmer in the millions before he even starts, farmers cannot afford to set aside their fields for a year in order to let the soil recoup lost minerals as God directed in the Old Testament. Every crop grown and harvested from farmers' fields takes out more and more of the precious nutrients—especially minerals—that are required to keep you healthy. Rather than allow the soil to recoup naturally, farmers add synthetic nutrients and chemicals—not so their crops are nutritious, but so they grow. As a result, the food you eat doesn't contain the amounts of nutrients you need. U.S. Senate document #264 states that our farm and range soils have been so depleted of minerals that the crops grown on these soils are mineral-deficient.

Even the government admits that food is not enough anymore. More than 99 percent of the U.S. population is deficient in trace minerals, according to U.S. Government document #249. To get the correct balance and amounts of minerals you need to supplement.

WHAT CAN HAPPEN
WITHOUT ENOUGH MINERALS?

Have you experienced muscle cramping, high blood pressure, or sudden weight gain? There are so many problems you can have if you don't get the right balance of minerals that you must supplement to be on the safe side. If you have high blood pressure, you should avoid salt, right?

That's not all there is to it. If you are deficient in potassium, any amount of salt will be a problem. Sudden weight gain can be caused by swelling, a very common symptom of mineral imbalances, or by eating too much (another symptom, believe it or not!). Muscle cramping can be caused by too much calcium, which should be balanced by three units of magnesium to every one of calcium. You need all the minerals in the correct proportions to avoid problems.

You are made of minerals. The collagen that plumps out your cheeks for a youthful look is fed by the mineral silica. Silica is found in the outer coverings of potatoes, green and red peppers, and cucumbers. Organic bean sprouts are also high in silica. Horsetail extract is a supplemental source of silica.

A lack of organic sulfur is linked to outbreaks of eczema. Organic sulfur, found in egg yolk, garlic, onions, cabbage, and horseradish, is an essential mineral necessary for healthy skin, hair, and nails. In any skin disorder, you can be pretty sure you're not getting enough of something.

The minerals calcium and magnesium are important to keeping your bones strong. Not enough selenium will cause profound muscle weakness, also known as Keshan's disease. Do you know someone with anorexia? This heart-wrenching eating disorder is associated with a deficiency of zinc.

WHAT ARE MINERALS
AND WHERE DO THEY COME FROM?

There are parts of the world where people eat clay in order to get dietary minerals. I kid you not! The syndrome is called pica. Eating clay is a symptom of a mineral deficiency. Some supplemental formulas get their minerals from clay, which is not a good idea. Clay tends to have too much aluminum and incorrect proportions of minerals. Instead, use clay packs on the skin. The minerals are lightly absorbed and can help clear skin conditions.

Minerals are mined naturally from rock, through erosion. The best mineral waters are those that flow through pristine rocky mountains, gathering minerals as they go. But even here, the amounts are not ideal for human consumption. Instead, take advantage of knowledgeable supplement manufacturers who use research to determine which minerals you need and how much.

Certain minerals are very important to the immune system. This is not to say you should take only these. But it helps to know what they are and how they are important. Make sure your mineral supplement has adequate amounts of these minerals.

ZINC

I told you about selenium in the antioxidant chapter. Like selenium, the mineral zinc is an antioxidant. This underestimated mineral is found to be deficient among people suffering from most degenerative diseases, especially those affecting cell DNA. The thymus gland, the traffic cop of the immune system, requires zinc in order to manufacture and secrete thymic hormones and protect the thymus against cellular damage. Low levels of both zinc and thymic hormones are prevalent in leukemia patients.

Zinc is a component of more than 200 enzymes and is needed for more body processes than any other mineral in the body. Many older people are marginally deficient in zinc, which means their immune system is compromised. A deficiency of zinc can lead to increased infections, poor wound healing, a decreased sense of taste or smell, and skin and eating disorders. Teenagers should know that not enough zinc can cause acne to get worse.

Are you trying to have a baby? Zinc is important for men to ensure healthy offspring. Zinc is found in high concentrations in the semen and is crucially important for proper functioning of DNA. Among populations exposed to radioactive fallout, studies show that those with enough zinc in their systems protected their offspring from bearing the mutagenic brunt of the impact. This was the finding of British researchers who discovered a high incidence of leukemia in children whose fathers have been exposed to external radiation before conception. Adequate zinc keeps metals out of the sex glands which attracts cell- and DNA-destroying radiation.

The recommended dosage (not RDA) is 15 milligrams.

COPPER

Most nutrients work in combinations. Zinc is balanced in the body by copper. Without it, zinc cannot be absorbed. Copper is important for bone strength, red and white blood cell growth, iron transport, cholesterol, blood sugar absorption, flexible blood vessels, and brain development. Copper is needed to activate the immune system's killer T cells. Even a marginal copper deficiency has been found in studies to inhibit T cell activity.

Do you have sallow, puffy skin, weak bones, arthritis, heart palpitations, fatigue, depression, or high cholesterol? You could be deficient in copper. A deficiency of the mineral copper has also been associated with aneurysms (ruptures of the artery) because copper is important for blood vessel strength and elasticity.

The recommended dosage is 2 to 3 milligrams. Foods high in copper are seafood, nuts, legumes (peas and beans), molasses, and raisins.

CHROMIUM

Chromium is extremely important to balance your blood sugar levels. Do you find yourself weak, faint, or nauseous if you haven't eaten? You could have low blood sugar. Diabetes and other blood sugar issues are on the increase, and one reason is the lack of chromium in today's diet. Chromium is a major regulator of insulin, and its deficiency in the body can be a leading factor in heart disease and diabetes. Diabetics are at greater risk of infection because they have impaired immune systems due to poor insulin efficiency and/or to a lack of insulin. Adequate levels of chromium not only protect the body against these two diseases but increase immune resistance to germ-caused disease and infections.

Chromium is found in parsley, real maple syrup, brewer's yeast, whole grains, mushrooms, and molasses.

MINERALS IN SOLUTION

Mineral tablets are very hard for the body to digest—only one to five percent absorbable. Since the process of digestion is a process of liquefaction, your body has to take a hard tablet and turn it into solution. This may not be possible due to a number of factors, such as inadequate stomach acid, stress, food allergies, and intestinal problems. If you want to be sure you get enough minerals from your supplement source, take them in solution. When they are in a liquid solution form, your body is better able to absorb and assimilate all of them.

For many years I have used Maximum Living's Mineral Rich, which is a tasty liquid mineral supplement that provides you with all the minerals, including trace minerals, your body needs, along with vitamins B12 and biotin . . . all in a delicious liquid that will be rapidly absorbed by your body. Thousands of people use this remarkable product daily to ensure their immune system is in peak fighting condition.

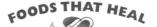

CHAPTER SIX

PRIME YOUR IMMUNE SYSTEM WITH EXERCISE AND AMINO ACIDS

> *Walking is an excellent exercise.*
> *At 65, my grandmother began*
> *walking five miles a day.*
> *She's now 100—and we have*
> *no idea where she is.*
>
> —Robert B. Reich

I TRIED TO GET A PLUMP FRIEND of mine to enroll in an aerobics class. "No. Absolutely not!" she exclaimed. "I tried that once." "What happened?" I asked. "I twisted, hopped, jumped, stretched, and pulled," she replied. "And by the time I got the stupid leotards on, the class was over!"

If you are overweight, does this mean your immune system is compromised? Let's just say it's not doing its best work. Your body should be a well-oiled machine. But if there is too much oil and dirt, it becomes sludge. Then you have diminished performance until your machine breaks down completely. Instead of waiting for this to happen, use only high octane fuel (good nutrition) and clean out the sludge through exercise, restoring it to top performance.

For your immune system to function at full peak, it needs to have all the advantages, including more oxygenated blood and more lean muscle mass than body fat. For lean muscle mass and oxygen, you need protein and exercise. But before you head to your local gym, take a moment and consider all the ways you can exercise for your health. You don't need aerobics classes, jogging, or bodybuilding workouts. Anything that makes you breathe a little harder and works the muscles will boost your immune system.

EASY ON THE EXERCISE

When it comes to optimal health, it is consistent, moderate exercise that makes the most difference to your immune system. According to a 1996 U.S. Surgeon General report, mild exercise is as beneficial as vigorous exercise. It may even be better, because there's less risk of injury. This is especially good news for people who are obese and find movement difficult.

When you think of exercise, do you think of aerobics, running, swimming, or tennis? These are vigorous activities intended to increase the supply of oxygen to the body (aerobic exercise means exercise "with oxygen"). You also exercise to build muscles, strengthen your heart, or lose weight by burning up calories. But you can achieve the same benefits with less work.

Oxygen plays a key role in your immune function. It is the source of the ammunition used by natural killer T cells against viruses and tumors. People who are ill or at risk for disease tend to exercise less, so there's less oxygen available to the body. This can prolong or make an illness worse.

Yoga uses focused breathing, muscle stretches, and relaxation to increase oxygen and strengthen muscles, including those of the heart. Focused breathing increases oxygen to all parts of the body. When you increase your oxygen intake, your blood flows better.

One of the reasons gentle exercise is so spectacularly effective is that it efficiently activates the lymph system, delivering immune cells from the lymph gland to where they are needed. This is not done efficiently when your body is pumped with adrenaline from stress.

Aerobics, swimming, and jogging can become more therapeutic by slowing them down and focusing on your breathing. Try this little experiment to see how slow exercise promotes well-being. Sit still for a minute. Focus on your breathing. Take slow easy breaths through your nose. Do this for a minute and see how much better you feel. This is exercising! Deepening the breath stimulates the lymph system and oxygenates the blood.

Walking is great because it exercises the internal organs.

The second factor that stimulates lymph circulation is movement—the act of contracting and releasing your muscles. But movement does not have to be vigorous to have a beneficial effect on your system. Simply lift your legs and arms or tighten and relax the muscles. A relaxing walk, pulling weeds, painting the fence, washing the car . . . just about any simple household chore qualifies as immune-boosting exercise. Now you have no excuse not to wash those windows!

AMINO ACIDS FOR ENERGY

The last time you were down with the flu, do you remember how tired and achy your muscles were? During illness, or when encountering an infection, one of the ways the immune system reacts is to use your body's protein for energy, sapping it of muscle strength in the process. Protein has to be replenished to avoid permanent damage, and this is where amino acids come in.

When you eat protein, digestive enzymes in the intestines break the proteins down into amino acids. When you are sick or exposed to illness, the body finds this difficult. Amino acids are absorbed into the bloodstream though the intestines and uses the amino acids as energy.

A healthy diet must also include each of the essential amino acids. Foods high in protein are also high in amino acids. These include meat, fish, cheese, poultry, and dairy products. A dietary protein that contains all ten essential amino acids is called a complete protein. Most animal proteins are complete, but many animal products also have high fat content. Most plant proteins are incomplete, so vegetarians must eat a variety of plant foods or use supplements to obtain all the essential amino acids. For meatless protein that is complete, combine whole grains with legumes (beans, peas, and lentils).

There approximately 22 amino acids that are components of protein. Eight of these cannot be manufactured by the body and must be supplied by food or supplementation. They are called free-form amino acids. Three of these are also antioxidants, further helping the body withstand the stresses of infection and illness. They are cysteine, glutathione, and methionine.

Cysteine and methionine combine to help rid the body of toxins and poisons. Methionine has been used successfully to treat Parkinson's disease. Adequate levels of methionine are credited with reduced levels of homocysteine. High homocysteine levels are associated with atherosclerosis, strokes, and osteoporosis. A lack of cysteine is directly correlated with AIDS and other immune-deficiency ailments, and cysteine has been used to treat patients with HIV-1 infection. Cysteine is important to lymph gland function and regulates several genes associated with the immune system.

Glutathione levels in the body are such a

strong predictor of immune health that it is used as a measurement. Researchers looking for nutrients that increase glutathione in the body determined that vitamin C and selenium increase levels. Researchers at the National Institutes of Health found that the immune cells of AIDS patients are glutathione deficient.

A COMPLETE AMINO ACID FORMULA

Amino acids are like the slats of a barrel. You need the full set, and one is only as effective as the shortest slat. For full supplemental benefit, look for a formula that includes all the free-form amino acids, such as Maximum Living's amino acid formula, which is all natural; derived from a hypoallergenic whey source.

Food allergies can interfere with the breakdown of protein and the production of amino acids, so you don't want them coming from your supplements! Specific non-essential amino acids are also included to provide additional support for your body's immune system.

For an excellent source of vegetable protein and amino acids, look for my favorite soy snack, "Maximum Living Nutrition Bites." It is packaged as chewy nuggets and comes in three flavors: chocolate, vanilla nut and peanut butter. The soy protein in these tasty snacks contains many other vital nutrients, including fiber and amino acids. Because they are natural, they have tryptophan, a serotonin precursor which helps depression and controls appetite.

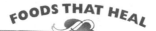
CHAPTER SEVEN

THERAPEUTIC HERBS FOR INFECTION CONTROL

> *The poorest man would not part*
> *with health for money,*
> *but the richest would gladly part*
> *with all their money for health.*
>
> —C. C. Colton

ONE OF THE REASONS we are losing the battle against infection and disease is that we've lost our roots—such as licorice root, ginger root, and goldenseal root.

There is much valuable healing information that our ancestors were aware of that has not been passed down to this generation. Fortunately for us, one root is still among us—the grassroots health food movement, which has progressed to legitimate science. Scientific studies are revealing the truth that many herbs and plants are of therapeutic and medicinal benefit to humans.

The use of herbs for medicinal purposes is centuries old, with centuries of documentation and experience to support their use. The success of herbs to treat infectious diseases has been forgotten, or pushed aside, in favor of profitable pharmaceuticals and unnatural antibiotics. As conventional medicine fails, people are turning to historically-proven remedies. Herbals have become so popular that patients are convincing their doctors to try them. Positive results compel even the most skeptical.

ECHINACEA

My friend Julie tells me that she learned the benefits of echinacea firsthand when her baby girl kept getting ear infections. Advice from the manager of a health food store prompted her to try an extract of echinacea and goldenseal, mixing a few drops in maple syrup when her daughter had a cold or runny nose. Her little girl is 11 years old today and has not had an ear infection since.

Echinacea is a natural herbal antibiotic that was one of the primary healing nutrients in the Nineteenth Century. It acts as an immune booster, fighting infection by killing microbes and increasing white blood cells. Research from Germany attests to its immunostimulant powers, especially for increasing the production of T-cells.

Before the advent of antibiotics, the herb was used to fight tuberculosis, diphtheria, malaria, sepsis, meningitis, gangrene, boils, carbuncles, and abscesses. It is particularly helpful when infections are accompanied by fevers.

In 1892, a Dr. Webster used echinacea to treat spinal meningitis in San Francisco. Following Webster's suggestions, other physicians of the time used its curative virtues to successfully treat meningitis and other convulsive and inflammatory disorders of the brain and spinal cord. This is particularly important in light of a new epidemic of antibiotic-resistant meningitis currently making the rounds in U.S. high schools.

Early in the 20th Century, doctors at Chicago's Cook County Hospital used echinacea to treat typhoid fever. Finley Ellingwood, M.D., recorded in his 1919 book, *The American Materia Medica, Therapeutics and Pharmacognosy*, that its use "effects an almost immediate stop in germ development." It was used at the hospital for years, with spectacular results during a time when whole populations were dying of typhoid.

Echinacea works best when accompanied by goldenseal, which also has anti-microbial properties.

GOLDENSEAL ROOT

In this country it was native Americans who first used goldenseal (hydrastis canadensis) to treat infection and inflammation. The generic name, hydrastis, is derived from two Greek words, "water" and "to accomplish," because of its beneficial effect on inflammations of the mucous membranes. The Cherokee introduced the plant with bright yellow roots to early American settlers. They used it as a wash for skin diseases, wounds, and for sore, inflamed eyes. Goldenseal root has acquired a considerable reputation as a natural antibiotic and as a remedy for urinary tract and fungus infections and Strep throat.

Numerous references to goldenseal began to appear in medical writings as far back as 1820 as a strong tea for indigestion. Try goldenseal tea the next time you have a stomachache or diarrhea. Not only does it kill bacterial infections, but it helps digest food.

Goldenseal contains an alkaloid called berberine that kills the bacterium Streptococcus and also prevents the attachment of Streptococcus to the throat. This is good news for parents when schools report outbreaks of Strep throat. Instead of waiting for it to get to your child, use goldenseal for prevention.

There's good news for women as well! The active ingredient in goldenseal, berberine, kills fungus and, combined with echinacea, works well against Candida albicans. Its astringent properties can also help control heavy menstrual bleeding.

THE KING OF BITTERS

King of Bitters is the common name for andrographis paniculata. Goldenseal is also a bitter. But don't let the name fool you. In this case, bitter is good. Bitters are herbs that have a bitter taste, ranging from the mildly bitter yarrow to the fiercely bitter rue. Angostura bitters, used by bartenders to make cocktails, was developed in 1824 by Dr. J. Siegert, who intended it for use as a tonic to treat fatigue and stomach ailments.

The taste of bitterness is transmitted by specific taste buds at the back of the tongue to the central nervous system, triggering a number of reflexes. These reflexes are important to digestion and immune system health. Bitters stimulate the flow of digestive juices, increasing the body's ability to break down food and increasing the appetite, important when sickness restricts your desire for nourishment. Bitters are thought to stimulate a range of liver activities, especially increasing the production and the release of bile from the gallbladder. Because bitters alter blood sugar, they can be helpful in the treatment of non-insulin dependent diabetes. But they are best known for detoxifying the liver and treating respiratory infections.

For centuries Asian medicine has used andrographis paniculata as a blood purifier to treat gastrointestinal tract and upper respiratory infections, fever, herpes, sore throat, and to cleanse the blood and liver. Today, in Scandinavian countries, it is used to prevent and treat common colds. Research conducted in the 1980s and 1990s has confirmed that it helps reduce fevers, fights bacteria and viruses, helps reduce blood sugar, reduces inflammation, acts as a pain killer, and helps clean and purify the blood and bowel.

IMMUNIZE NATURALLY WITH M-U BOOST

Now that you know what to look for, let me tell you where to find it. Maximum Living's M-U

Boost formula includes the above-described herbs and adds the antioxidant mineral selenium, zinc, and alpha lipoic acid for a power-packed one-two and even three punch against infection.

CHAPTER EIGHT

FLAVONOIDS—4,000 COLORFUL REASONS TO EAT FRUITS AND VEGETABLES

Eighty-two percent of people know that a poor diet can increase their risk of cancer. 15 percent of people have changed their diet to lower their risk of cancer.

—*Hippocrates magazine*

WE COMPARE "apples to oranges" to show that two things are very different. But in this case apples and oranges have something in common. They're both good sources of flavonoids—a group of nutrients found in fruits, vegetables, and herbs as well as in tea and red wine. The most beneficial flavonoids are found in the most colorful fruits and vegetables. They occur in high concentrations in the juice and peel of citrus fruits, onions, grapes and grape juice, papaya, broccoli, apricots, Swiss chard, persimmons, green tea, soy products, cherries, berries, and grains, especially buckwheat.

There are 12 subcategories and approximately 4,000 different flavonoids identified to date. A simple definition describes flavonoids as "any group of substances found in fruits and vegetables essential for processing vitamin C and needed to maintain capillary walls." Their impressive health-giving qualities include the ability to reduce inflammation, prevent bruising, retard cancer, battle infection, increase circulation, fight pain and strengthen bones.

PROVEN HEALTH BENEFITS

Finnish researchers accessed diet information that had been collected on more than 10,000 people in the late 1960s and early 1970s. Using modern food composition tables, they calculated the flavonoid content of the foods the people were eating and then compared their later incidences of chronic diseases. The people who ate the most of several common flavonoids were about 20 percent less likely than others in the study to suffer from heart disease or stroke, and about 35 percent less likely to develop asthma. In men, high flavonoid intake was also linked to a reduced risk of lung and prostate cancer.

Most of the flavonoids measured came from seven types of foods: apples, oranges, white cabbage, onions, grapefruit, berries, and juices.

BIOFLAVONOIDS FOR THE BODY

"Bioflavonoids" are used interchangeably with

"flavonoids." However, not all flavonoids affect the health of the body. The term "bioflavonoids" signify those that biologically influence the body. In other words, all bioflavonoids are flavonoids, but not all flavonoids are bioflavonoids. To make it clear that I am talking about natural chemicals that encourage a healthy body, I will henceforth refer to them as bioflavonoids.

Some facts about bioflavonoids: vitamin C relies on them to work, so always choose a vitamin C supplement that includes, ideally, citrus bioflavonoids. Citrus bioflavonoids boost the health-giving qualities of vitamin C. They are also credited with keeping toxins, such as those in cigarette smoke, from mutating normal cells into cancer cells.

My home state of California may have gotten the message that secondhand smoke is hazardous to our health, but many other states and European countries still allow smoking in all public areas. To protect myself, I never travel without my Maximum Living Solu-C with green tea. It combines the health-giving bioflavonoids rutin, quercetin, and green tea with vitamin C to protect me against being ravaged by clouds of chemicals.

Rutin, found in buckwheat, helps increase capillary strength and ensures fast healing. It's a great help for varicose veins and bruising from sitting for hours in cramped airplane seats.

Quercetin has been shown in studies to be particularly helpful in the fight against phlebitis, the inflammation of the veins that can lead to blockages. It has also been found to help allergy symptoms and fight flu viruses—another important factor when flying in close quarters with sick people.

The bioflavonoids in green tea inhibit the growth of the dangerous bacterium staphylococcus, which is blamed for many unnecessary and tragic hospital deaths.

Soybeans contain genistein and daidzein, powerful antioxidants and cancer inhibitors that lower the risks for breast and prostate cancer.

Grapeseed extract (one of the proanthocyanidins—a type of bioflavonoid and a potent anti-inflammatory) strengthens capillaries and prevents the inflammation believed to cause strokes and heart disease.

Curcumin, in the form of the spice turmeric, has been used in both the Indian and Chinese systems of medicine for the treatment of many forms of inflammation. Its anti-inflammatory properties are likened to the pharmaceutical effects of hydrocortisone and phenylbutazone, only much safer. It is the curcumin which gives tumeric its yellow color, that has been found in studies to work better than even ibuprofen, a popular over-the-counter pain medicine. In one study on rats, researchers found 20 mg of curcumin worked as well as 200 mg of ibuprofen. And unlike ibuprofen, no toxic effects have been reported.

Bromelain, found naturally in pineapple, has been used in the treatment of cancer. Its ability to reduce swelling and inflammation means it can help with lowering blood pressure, arthritis, joint and muscle pain, ulcer healing, and any kind of infection. Bromelain is also an enzyme, leading us to another chapter and another category of immune boosters.

A FANTASTIC REASON TO BUY ORGANIC

Fruits and vegetables grown without synthetic chemicals have higher levels of flavonoids than produce treated with chemicals, according to a provocative new study by researchers at the University of California, Davis. Food scientists compared corn, blackberries, and strawberries and found that those grown without synthetic chemical pesticides had consistently more flavonoids. Another thing they noted was that frozen fruit and vegetables retained their flavonoids better than fresh. This is not surprising. Once a fruit or vegetable is picked, time diminishes its nutritional value. When frozen fresh off the vine, fresh foods retain their values.

A FANTASTIC REASON
TO GROW YOUR OWN FOOD

You've already learned that farm soil is nourished with synthetic chemicals and protected from pests by synthetic pesticides. Farm soil is also deficient in nutrients. When you add that to the amount of time from the field to your dinner table, you realize that even fresh isn't fresh anymore, and what should be the healthiest food isn't always the case. Buying organic food helps, but for optimum impact and performance from your diet, grow food at home. A window box of herbs, a fruit tree, zucchini squash, tomatoes or carrots . . . anyone can grow something—even you! See how good fresh grown food tastes.

My mother was planting seeds one afternoon when I dropped by to visit. As I gazed at her not-too-straight rows, I suggested that she mark each row so that she would know what she had planted. Without hesitation she replied, "My dear girl, this is a garden, not a cemetery. I expect all of these seeds to come up and identify themselves."

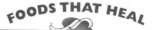

CHAPTER NINE

PROTECT YOUR INNER SANCTUM WITH "GOOD GUY" BACTERIA AND ENZYMES

*Health is not valued
till sickness comes.*

—*Thomas Fuller*

I WAS PARTICIPATING in an important conference on the effects of chemicalized food, and the speaker was addressing the audience.

"The food we eat today is dangerous to our health. Red meat contains hormones, injected chemicals, and saturated fat; the high amount of phosphorus in soft drinks depletes calcium, magnesium, and other strategic minerals; processed food is loaded with carcinogens, and none of us realizes the long-term harm caused by the germs in our drinking water.

"But there is one thing that is the most dangerous

of all, and we all have, or will, eat it. Can anyone here tell me what food it is that causes the most grief and suffering for years after eating it?"

A 75-year-old man in the front row stood up and answered, "Is it wedding cake?"

THE BAD GUYS

There isn't one food that affects everyone the same, but there are many forms of bacteria that make us sick. The bioterrorism connection to anthrax (bacillus anthracis) will be discussed in the next chapter, but most anthrax infections historically occur after the bacterium from contaminated meat, wool, hides, or leather enters a cut in the skin. When the bacterium is ingested, it acts similar to food poisoning, but can also include vomiting blood and bloody diarrhea.

Found in raw or undercooked chicken, Campylobacter is one of the most common causes of traveler's diarrhea. It is of special concern to the military because it affects 20 to 30 percent of military personnel deployed overseas.

Stomach cancer and ulcers are caused by Helicobacter pylori, found in more than 90 percent of peptic ulcer patients.

Other bacterial enemies are bacteria staphylococci (the staph infection common in hospitals), streptococci (Strep throat), clostridium botulinum (botulism or food poisoning), Escherichia coli (E. coli), and another common food bacterial sickness, salmonella.

THE FACTS OF BACTERIA LIFE

What most people don't understand is that we are supposed to have bacteria in our bodies. Certain kinds are both normal and helpful. That's why antibiotics can be harmful. They kill all the bacteria—good and bad. It's not the bacteria that are the problem, but the kind of bacteria.

A healthy human gastrointestinal tract contains almost 100 different species and a total of 100 trillion bacteria, referred to as intestinal flora. When the normal balance of these bacteria is disturbed by illness or antibiotics, the most common effect is diarrhea. Cramping, gas, and pain are also symptoms of an unbalanced system.

How do you know you are deficient in good bacteria? You know when the bad bacteria are able to make you sick. Just because someone hands you bad bacteria in a burrito doesn't mean you'll get sick. You'll get sick if something—antibiotics, stress, or another illness—has minimized your intestinal army to a point where they can no longer hold the defensive line.

For decades health experts have scratched their heads over bacteria that harms no one in a native population but knocks tourists off their feet. Why, if they make visitors sick, don't the bacteria also cause illness in the people living there? Because the stress of travelling has undermined the immune system and because tourists pick up bacteria that are alien to their systems.

THE GOOD GUYS

Probiotics are the good bacteria. They work by colonizing the small intestine and crowding out pathogenic (disease-causing) bacteria, restoring balance to the intestinal flora, and stimulating the body's immune system.

The good guys have long names but bear with me. You need to know this. Most of us have heard of lactobacillus acidophilus, a bacteria used to culture yogurt and milk. It cultures more than yogurt. It also cultures human health. In test tube experiments, acidophilus inhibited the growth of 27 different types of bacteria, 10 of which are common disease-causers. Traveler's diarrhea has been reduced with a mixture of lactobacillus acidophilus, lactobacillus bulgaricus, bifidobacterium, and streptococcus thermophilus.

Probiotics have been used for many other conditions, including milk allergies, irritable bowel syndrome, Crohn's disease, respiratory and GI problems resulting from cystic fibrosis, cancer prevention, high cholesterol, tuberculosis, eczema, canker sores, and vaginal and urinary tract infections. They can help with gas, cramps, food allergies, colon problems, and have been found safe for even young children (in dosages designed for them).

One of the ways that bacteria boost the immune system is by creating enzymes. And one of the ways you can charge your infection fighting machinery is by supplementing with enzymes as well as probiotic bacteria.

DIGESTIVE ENZYMES

There are two kinds of enzymes. The first are digestive. They are taken to help break down food and are designed to dissolve in the stomach. They also diminish with age, causing the problems we typically associate with age, such as weight gain, constipation, arthritis, and heart disease.

Examples of digestive enzymes are protease, which digests protein; amylase, which digests carbohydrates; and lipase, which digests fats. People allergic to milk (lactose intolerant) lack the enzyme lactase, which breaks down milk sugar. If you have this insufficiency, you can supplement with lactobacillus acidophilus, which makes the necessary lactase in the intestine, or you can supplement with the enzyme lactase.

You can tell you lack digestive enzymes when your food sits in your stomach like an anchor on a cruise ship. Or you experience gas and indigestion after eating. Alpha-galactosidase is an enzyme that can be taken to avoid the gaseous side effect of eating beans and other legumes. It is sold under the brand name Beano.

Incomplete digestion, caused by a lack of digestive enzymes, creates an internal environment that invites disease and infection. It's not a pretty picture when undigested food sits and putrefies in your body. Bad bacteria then proliferates, overpowering even your best immune defenses.

ENTERIC-COATED ENZYMES

Enteric-coated, or metabolic, enzymes are coated so they pass through the stomach and are absorbed in the intestine and bloodstream. Once in the bloodstream, they are able to fight disease.

Enzymes are so important for good health that for a good part of the Twentieth Century, European oncologists have included enzyme therapy as a natural, non-toxic therapy against cancer. Almost all the leading alternative cancer specialists who treat Americans prescribe both digestive enzymes and enteric-coated enzyme supplements as primary or adjuvant cancer therapies. Called "systemic enzyme therapy," enteric-coated enzymes mimic the benefits of enzyme-packed food, such as fresh fruits and vegetables, preventing the chronic inflammation that promotes illness and disease. Enzymes break up debris in an injured area, decrease swelling, and stimulate the body's own natural enzymatic processes without causing the immune system to be suppressed (as occurs when cortisone is used to fight inflammation).

Enzymes also keep trophoblast cells in check, preventing their overgrowth and mutation, which contributes to uterine fibroids, heart disease, endometriosis, fibrocystic breasts, ovarian tumors and cancer. In cases of cancer, blood circulating enzymes de-shield the cancer cell, allowing the body's natural defense system to recognize it as a foreign invader and destroy it. Blood circulating enzymes also work for fibrocystic disease (breast, uterine fibroids, ovarian cysts, etc.) because they digest scar tissue.

ENZYMES FROM FRUITS AND VEGETABLES

Studies and experts agree that the bodies of people who eat the most fruits and vegetables have the most natural enzymes and dramatically reduced levels of cancer and other diseases. Digestive organs, such as the pancreas and liver, produce most of the body's digestive enzymes, while the remainder should come from uncooked foods, such as fresh fruit and vegetables, raw sprouted grains, seeds and nuts, unpasteurized dairy products, and enzyme supplements.

Eating food in its natural, unprocessed state is vital to the maintenance of good health, and a lack of it in the modern diet is directly responsible for degenerative disease. The cooking of food, particularly if heat is prolonged and over 118 degrees, such as when food is fried, destroys enzymes. This is why by the time we reach middle age we become metabolically depleted of enzymes. The glands and major organs, including the brain, suffer the most from a deficiency. The brain may actually shrink as a result of a cooked, over-refined diet devoid of enzymes.

I venture to guess that our country's high rates of obesity and heart disease are directly connected with eating less fruits and vegetables. Although whales have up to six inches of fat keeping them warm, their arteries are unclogged. Similarly, Eskimos, who frequently eat large quantities of fat, are often not obese. Both these groups eat the fat-digesting enzyme lipase in the form of raw foods.

HEALTH-GIVING SUPPLEMENTAL FORMULAS

Maximum Living distributes two excellent enzyme formulas: Multi-Enzyme, with all the digestive enzymes necessary to properly assimilate food, and Enzyme-Ease, an enterically-coated enzyme supplement that includes pancreatin, a pancreatic enzyme.

God promises we will be healed and I believe Him. The God who loves us infinitely cares about our deepest needs. He comforts us in grief, provides for our needs and heals our diseases.

Beloved, I wish above all things
that thou mayest prosper
and be in health,
even as thy soul prospereth.

—3 John 2

CHAPTER TEN

SHOULD WE WORRY ABOUT THE THREAT OF BIOTERRORISM?

So do not fear, for I am with you;
do not be dismayed, for I am
your God. I will strengthen you
and help you; I will uphold you
with my righteous right hand.

—Isaiah 41:10

I RELY ON THIS VERSE from the prophet Isaiah in every area of my life. It lifts my anxiety immediately when I realize that it is a sin to be dismayed because we are doubting God's ability to take care of any situation. Nevertheless, we must still prepare and use the knowledge we have gained in this book to heighten our immune systems to super immunity so they are impervious to super bugs, viruses, and bacteria, whether they be smallpox, Ebola virus, bubonic plague, botulism, anthrax, or, the newest addition to our list of plagues: Severe Acute Respiratory Syndrome (SARS), a highly contagious respiratory virus from Asia.

Your most important defense is for you to be knowledgeable. The Bible also says, "My people perish for lack of knowledge." The Centers for Disease Control has identified over 40 agents as potential bioterrorism threats. Our new world of horrors includes not only anthrax letters and passenger planes crashing into skyscrapers but also dirty bombs, poison gas, suicide bombings, and terrorist operatives injected with smallpox virus and sent to America to infect as many people as possible.

Forewarned is forearmed. These are the most likely potential bioterrorism weapons that we must guard against:

- Smallpox—virus
- Bubonic Plague—bacteria
- Anthrax—bacteria

As you can see, two of the three are bacterial threats. Read over the hygiene and probiotics chapters to learn about preventing bacterial infections. There are several helpful supplements discussed in the herb chapter to help you prevent and overcome viral infections. And, to better prepare you to identify the threats, these are their signs and symptoms.

SMALLPOX

Unfortunately, smallpox still lingers as a potential biological warfare threat and is maintained in at least two laboratories in the United States and Russia. With the dismantling of the Russian biological warfare research program, it is not inconceivable that disgruntled former scientists took biological weapons with them and/or were bought off by other countries to produce weapons for them. A *60 Minutes* investigation found that Saddam Hussein acquired smallpox virus from a laboratory in Russia. Russian scientists have been helping countries such as Iran and Iraq develop biological weapons.

In the book, Catastrophe, Clinton's Role in America's Greatest Disaster, Colonel Byron Weeks, M.D., considers smallpox to be a likely biological weapon used against the United States because those previously vaccinated have largely lost immunity and because of intelligence knowledge of extensive research programs conducted by Russia and Iraq.

The early stages of smallpox are so similar to chicken pox that, if you didn't have the information here, chances are it would not be diagnosed right away, especially since cases haven't been seen since the mid 1970s. Once exposed, the incubation period is about 12 days. Initial symptoms include high fever, fatigue, and head and back aches. A characteristic rash, most prominent on the face, arms, and legs, follows in 2 to 3 days. The rash starts with flat red lesions that evolve at the same rate. Lesions become pus-filled after a few days and then begin to crust early in the second week. Scabs develop and then separate and fall off after about 3 to 4 weeks. Death may occur in up to 30 percent of cases.

In the majority of cases, smallpox is spread from one person to another by infected saliva droplets. People with smallpox are most infectious during the first week of illness, because that is when the largest amount of virus is present in saliva. However, some risk of transmission lasts until all the scabs have fallen off. Contaminated clothing or bed linen can also spread the virus.

BUBONIC PLAGUE

When we think of this virus, spread by rat fleas and unsanitary conditions, we think of history, before the use of antibiotics and handwashing. Plague outbreaks have killed about 200 million people in the past 1,500 years. The most infamous, Europe's Black Death, started in 1347, killing 25 million people in Europe and 13 million in the Middle East and China within five years. At its worst, the bubonic plague killed two million victims a year.

The virus is alive and well in this country today. Bubonic plague is active in about 15 American states and occurs in 1,000 to 3,000 people worldwide each year, according to the Centers for Disease Control and Prevention. The disease occurs in 10 to 20 people each year in the United States—mostly in rural areas of the West. About one in seven U.S. cases is fatal.

The most recent case was November 2002. Two tourists were hospitalized in New York City after they likely contracted bubonic plague in their home state of New Mexico. Rodents and fleas on the couple's New Mexico property tested positive for plague.

The symptoms of Bubonic Plague include high fever and swollen, painful lymph nodes, called "buboes."

ANTHRAX

It's what we know that can hurt us. Kevin G. Briggs, current director of the U.S. Disaster Preparedness Institute, said that we know Iraq has hidden and lied about much of its biological warfare program. It has admitted testing anthrax and other agents as part of its program. And we know that anthrax weapons can be produced with the same killing capacity as nuclear weapons for the fraction of the cost and expertise.

Former Secretary of Defense William Cohen stated that a five-pound bag of anthrax, if properly dispersed, could kill half the population of Washington, D.C. If ingested in a sufficient dose, an intestinal form of anthrax could kill somewhere between 25 and 60 percent of those infected.

Anthrax can be contracted from the skin (cutaneous), inhaled through the mouth and nose (inhalational), or by eating contaminated meat (gastrointestinal). The last cases of accidental infections (assuming the most recent cases were premeditated) were in the 1970s. Of some comfort is the knowledge that anthrax cannot be spread from person to person.

Historically, most anthrax infections occur after the bacterium from contaminated meat, wool, hides, or leather enters a cut in the skin. The incubation period ranges from 1 to 12 days. It begins as a skin infection; first a raised bump that looks like a spider bite, then a painless ulcer with dying (black) tissue in the center. Only about 20 percent of people with cutaneous anthrax will die from it.

The most lethal type of exposure is when inhaled (inhalational). It is estimated that 75 percent will die from the exposure. Anthrax spores must be distributed through an aerosol. Studies show that 4,000 to 5,000 spores must be present to cause an infection. The incubation period of inhalational anthrax among humans is unclear, but it is reported to range from 1 to 7 days, possibly ranging up to 60 days. It resembles a viral respiratory illness, and initial symptoms include sore throat, mild fever, muscle aches, and malaise. These symptoms may progress to respiratory failure and shock with meningitis frequently developing.

The symptoms of gastrointestinal anthrax are similar to food poisoning, but can also include vomiting blood and bloody diarrhea.

A NEW VIRUS CALLED SARS

Severe acute respiratory syndrome (SARS) is a respiratory illness that has been reported in Asia, North America, and Europe. When SARS first came on the scene we didn't know what hit us. All researchers knew was that it came from Asia and spread from there.

The medical establishment needed something to go on, so they established guidelines for diagnosis. You are suspected of having SARS if you have a body temperature greater than 100.4°F and at least one of the following: cough, shortness of breath or difficulty breathing. And if you have travelled within 10 days of onset of symptoms to an area with documented or suspected community transmission of SARS such as China, Hong Kong, Hanoi, Vietnam, Singapore and Toronto, Canada. Or you have had close contact within 10 days of onset of symptoms with a person suspected to have SARS.

The same immune boosting therapies can be used to prevent SARS. But conventional medicine does not know this. What they do know is that their storehouse of antibiotics don't work against it.

SARS is spread like a cold or flu virus, by close, person-to-person contact. Most cases of SARS have involved people who cared for or lived with someone with SARS, or had direct contact with infectious material (for example, respiratory secretions) from a person who has SARS. Potential ways in which SARS can be spread include touching the skin of other people or objects that are contaminated with infectious droplets and then touching your eye(s), nose, or mouth. This can happen when someone who is sick with SARS coughs or sneezes droplets onto themselves, other people, or nearby surfaces. It also is possible that SARS can be spread more broadly through the air or by other ways that are currently not known. It is always possible that, if isolated, the virus can be used by terrorists.

I believe the battle against SARS is not as difficult as some think. This first occurred to me as I was watching television news images of Beijing health officials hosing down the sidewalks and back alleys of the teeming Chinese capital with bleach. I recalled that dog breeders, when confronted with an epidemic of the deadly Parvo virus that threatens to kill newborn puppies, will use diluted bleach to rid the environment of the threat.

Bleach—sodium hypochlorite—has been used for years as a folk remedy for mouth/throat infections in parts of North America. It kills germs and viruses because it releases atomic oxygen (like ozone for swimming pools). Vitamin C, in high amounts such as 20-30 grams, also releases atomic oxygen. At this amount it becomes oxidative instead of antioxidative, and can thus effectively kill bacteria and viruses.

Now, I'm not advocating that people drink bleach, even diluted 20-1, but in the absence of vitamin C supplementation, and threatened with a deadly virus, I might try anything.

VACCINATIONS REQUIRE CAUTION

Everything we are told about biological weapons leads us to believe that, once infected with a virus or bacteria, there is little hope of a complete recovery. Even if you survive the infection, you are left with scars or disability.

Dr. Ken Alibek, a medical doctor with a Ph.D. in microbiology, was once lead scientist in the former Soviet Union's biological weapons program. He defected to the United States in 1992 and wrote a book entitled *Biohazard*, describing how the Soviets hatched smallpox virus in chicken eggs and cooked anthrax into fluffy powders for easy dissemination.

Your best hope is preventing infection through immune system boosting. Alibek believes that the body's immune system has a natural capacity to defend itself, even from the deadliest virus. He believes research into what he calls "biodefense," is far more promising than "attempts to rig office buildings and public monuments with detection devices or to stockpile vaccines."

Vaccinations have, in the past, been the first line of defense. And most rely on them. But never take it for granted that problems won't occur. Take smallpox, for example. Until 1972, the vaccine was routinely given. However, what wasn't commonly known was that the vaccine was killing more people than the infection.

The last outbreak of smallpox in the U.S. occurred in 1947 when Eugene LeBar, a 47-year-old merchant, arrived by bus to New York City from Mexico City carrying the virus. Twelve people contracted the virus; two of them died. Three died as a result of the vaccine.

Ronald Atlas, president of the American Society for Microbiology and a bioterrorism expert, estimates that 1,000 people would die if the country as a whole were to be inoculated. To complicate matters, the infection caused by the vaccine is contagious. The sore that forms at the site of the shot fills with live viruses. People in the past were known to accidentally spread the infection on their own bodies or to someone else by touching the sore and then touching someone or something else. Or someone else—especially babies and toddlers—would touch the sore. In Atlas' scenario of 1,000 fatalities, 200 of those deaths would occur among people who caught the virus from someone who recently received the shot.

Beyond complications, the 1947 outbreak demonstrated another truth about the vaccine: It doesn't confer lifelong immunity. LeBar had been vaccinated as a child and received a booster the year before he left Mexico, which evidently didn't "take."

Participants at an international symposium on pertussis—the whooping cough vaccine—concluded that the current whole-cell pertussis vaccine can cause a wide spectrum of permanent brain damage, ranging from learning disabilities to severe retardation to seizure disorders.

A distrust of vaccinations is healthy as none are always safe. While most children can tolerate them, vaccinations can harm children in several ways. Live virus vaccines can produce the infection that the vaccine is supposed to prevent. For example, live polio should never be administered to a child who comes in contact with an HIV patient. The virus can "leap" to the HIV patient and produce polio. Reports exist of previously healthy parents who have developed polio from the viral vaccine given to their children.

A second opportunity for damage comes from neurotoxic materials sometimes found in vaccines. A full generation of children in America were injected with dangerous doses of highly toxic ethyl mercury from 1990 through 2000, a major ingredient in a chemical called Thimersol, an additive and biological preservative packaged into multi-dose vials of many childhood vaccines. With each dose of vaccine that contained Thimerosal, a child would also get an injection of toxic mercury in excess of the federal government's own safety guidelines.

The third way that vaccines can cause damage is through allergic reactions and the development of an autoimmune response, stimulated by the vaccine and its adjuvant. Vaccines always contain adjuvants, which are substances known to amplify the body's response to the vaccine. These adjuvants are known to cause allergic and autoimmune responses on their own.

The simplistic view that we, the patient, are the victim and the infectious agent is the villain rejects the personal responsibility we have in defending ourselves. We are not helpless to make a difference. We are powerful. Armed with the knowledge found in this book and your cornucopia of nutritional supplement options, for the first time in history you have the power to enact serious vengeance against the bugs and viral villains that threaten to plague you.

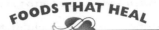

NUTRITIONAL SUPPLEMENT OPTIONS

THERE IS A REASON I recommend Maximum Living Supplements. For many years I have been involved with the formulation of their leading-edge products based on the latest scientific research and highest production standards to ensure the natural force and power of the nutrients are retained. Just as fruits and vegetables can be low in nutrition when grown in poor soil, so can the sources for nutritional supplements.

The plant sources for Maximum Living products are meticulously chosen—usually one in seven—for their high nutritional values. I've been to the manufacturing plant and know that the scientists there spend painstaking hours evaluating the raw materials used for their formulas.

And because I am dedicated to the protection and enrichment of my body and the need to protect myself against the effects of skin- and body-degrading free radicals, I choose Maximum Living's antioxidant formula.

I know that the best supplement formula uses living food: freeze-dried sprouts, vegetables, and herbals for the full spectrum of vital B vitamins, important to a healthy nervous system. This is why I recommend, and take, Maximum Living's Vita Sprout.

For many years I have used and recommended Maximum Living's Mineral Rich, which is a delicious liquid in solution; the most highly absorbable form of mineral supplement that provides you with all the minerals, including trace minerals, your body needs, along with vitamins B12, biotin, and silica for beautiful hair and nails. The liquid in solution aspect encourages your body to fully utilize the health-giving benefits of minerals in the fastest and most efficient manner possible.

For the full supplemental benefit of all the free-form amino acids necessary for optimum immune system energy and strong muscles, target Maximum Living's amino acid formula.

Maximum Living's M-U Boost formula includes the virus-fighting herbs echinacea, goldenseal, and andrographis paniculata, and adds the antioxidant minerals selenium and zinc as well as alpha lipoic acid for a power-packed punch against infection.

To protect myself against chemicals and germs present in the environment and in public places, I never travel without my Maximum Living Solu-C with green tea. It combines the health-giving bioflavonoids rutin, quercetin, and green tea with vitamin C.

For your digestive army of enzyme helpers

and your battle against bacterial bad guys, Maximum Living distributes two excellent enzyme formulas: Multi-Enzyme, with all the digestive enzymes necessary to properly assimilate food, and Enzyme-Ease, an enterically-coated enzyme for bloodstream battles against systemic infections and disease.

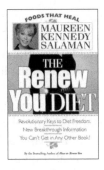

Also in this Series

#620 / $7.95

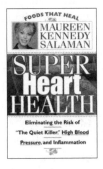

Also in this Series

#625 / $7.95

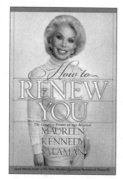
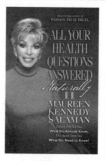
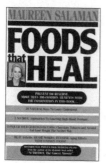

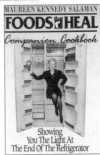
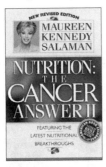
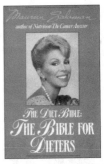